sex
education
and the new
morality

sex
education
and the new
morality

a search for a meaningful social ethic

 child study association of america
distributed by the columbia university press

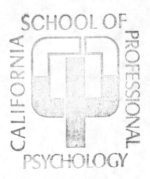

Proceedings of the 42nd Annual Conference, March 7, 1966, Child Study Association of America
9 East 89th Street, New York, N. Y. 10028

contents

introduction

In this century we have witnessed dramatic changes in our knowledge and understanding of the significance of sexuality in the total growth of children. Today most parents and professional people affirm the value of imparting to children factual information and positive feelings about sex which are appropriate to their interest and ability to understand.

When considering the sexual attitudes and behavior of the adolescent, however, responsible adults seem to feel somewhat confused. At every level of society, boys and girls, young men and women, appear to be rejecting previously-determined standards of sexual conduct. We are understandably concerned about the so-called sexual revolution which appears to result in an increase of promiscuity, unwanted pregnancies, early and unsatisfactory marriages, abortion and incidence of venereal disease. However, some by-products of this revolution have also been good: a greater freedom to discuss sexual questions, and a lessening of the inhibiting fears of sexual expression. Nevertheless, we still seem to have less assurance about what approaches to adopt, what to tell young people in order to help them develop a healthy basic value system for themselves.

The 1966 conference of The Child Study Association of America was devoted to this all-pervasive, complex subject of sexual behavior, sex education, and social ethics, which concerns everyone whose interest and responsibility is helping individuals and families. The participants were drawn from the fields of psychiatry, social work, education for social work, teacher education, the arts, and religious education. Discussions and questions focussed on sexuality and its relationship to personal identity, the impact of social forces on the development of sexual attitudes and behavior today, and how young people themselves feel about these matters. Mr. Dore Schary comments on "The Arts and the Sexual Image,"—a provocative look at what we ourselves reflect to youth in our culture. The panel discussion, in a lively, controversial fashion, probes the factors which we need to understand in developing a new approach to sex education—an approach which will be relevant and meaningful to young people today.

You will not find here a few easy lessons on how to deal with problems of sex education. However, we believe that you will find much in this report that will open new avenues of thought, that will enlighten and stimulate. The Association is deeply grateful to all the participants in the conference for making this volume possible.

A. D. BUCHMUELLER
Executive Director

sexuality and its implications for personal identity and fulfillment

MORTON S. EISENBERG, M.D.

■ The life situations in which a young person can experiment toward becoming an adult, as well as the totality of childhood experiences that shape his destiny, differ widely from individual to individual, and from one part of our society to another. All these factors will influence adolescence in the form of its expression. Nevertheless, the broad interaction between the biological, the psychological and the social aspects of adolescence—for that is my frame of reference—has general application.

I shall not attempt to establish an ethic of sexual behavior. Psychology and sociology can only study morality; they cannot decide what society ought to consider as "good" or "bad" behavior. Although investigation of morality does influence such decisions, it does not arbitrate them. The fact that sexual morality can be a subject for discussion in such an open public forum as this, is in itself indicative of the change that has occurred in our attitude toward sexuality. When

Dr. Eisenberg is a psychoanalyst, and a member of the faculty, Columbia School of Social Work.

many of us were adolescents such a discussion as this would have been inconceivable, or at least shocking. It would be no less absurd to label this event anti-moral than it would be to assume that adolescent sexual behavior and the changing social code of the youth of our society is anti-moral—but I will have more to say about this shortly.

We are hindered in our efforts to gain some perspective on this subject because it is overcast with an intensity of emotion and confusion that is the usual consequence of the collision between the older generation and the younger generation. It is a collision that has its roots in the complex changes that take place when our children reach this stage of transition between childhood and adulthood.

In primitive societies, with the onset of puberty, young boys or girls were conducted with elaborate "rites of passage" into adulthood. Their predetermined roles of wife, mother, husband, hunter, warrior, worker, were assumed with little delay. In different historical eras, e.g., before the industrial revolution and even through the first part of our own century, when the speed of change was slower, young people gradually assumed commitment to the responsibilities of adulthood—work, marriage and children, within the supportive confines of a larger family unit wherein the experience of the several generations was similar.

Today it is even impossible for parents to help their children with third grade arithmetic. Under these earlier conditions, the uncertainties, conflicts and fears preliminary to an adolescent's development of an adult sense of personal identity, were seldom present.

On the other hand, in our rapidly changing society

where occupational choice requires lengthy preparation, where social role is uncertain, and commitment to a sexual mate is deferred, the young boy and girl must set forth from the familiar and relatively comfortable shores of their childhood into a land that is new and strange. The contours of this strange land are constantly in flux—beset by forces acting upon it from many directions. The most decisive of these forces is the result of advancing biological maturity. The awakening of the endocrine system, an event predetermined by an innate genetic timetable, will within a few years transform the body of the young boy and girl into that of a sexually mature man and woman.

These biological changes bring in their wake profound psychological consequences. Above all there is a vast increase in the intensity of the sexual drives, bringing with them a dramatic end to the quiescence of the latency period, and a disruption of the personality organization of childhood.

Psychoanalysis has shown that adult sexuality is a force that has its archaic expression in the dim history of one's life. In the course of development from infancy to adulthood, the pleasure-seeking activities motivated by this force change according to an inborn biological schedule, culminating in the mature sexual needs existing between a man and a woman.

However, unlike other genetically determined maturational events, the evolution of sexuality is highly influenced by the growing child's relationships with its parents. The course of development of sexuality and morality is very much rooted in the lengthy dependency of the human infant on his parents, and especially in the early months of life, on his mother. She is the ultimate source of his frustration, his pleasure and his survival.

There is a great deal we do not understand about the nature of the communication between a mother and her baby in these early months. Nevertheless, we do know that the child's total experiences of frustration and pleasure within the matrix of this uniquely human tie, form a bridge to another human being and to the world outside of himself. It is within this bond that the core of his sense of himself as a separate entity, and the foundation of his ability to love, first take shape. We also know that because of this intense tie between a mother and her baby, her attitudes will enhance or discourage certain kinds of responses. This is true not only in the immediate sense, but also in the sense in which she transmits the cultural expectations of her society.

Throughout childhood the young boy or girl takes into his expanding self traits, qualities, values, ideals—positive and negative—after the model of his parents, or rather his perception of them. This internal model is a crucial factor in the identity system of childhood. Around the third or fourth year of his life, this process of identity formation is catalyzed further by the maturing of his sexuality. As the sexual drive becomes centered in his genital organs, he makes a startling and disconcerting discovery about his body: He discovers his sexual identity.

The child receives support for the establishment of his sexual identity from the emphasis that his parents place on various masculine and feminine characteristics. More important than this, however, is the degree to which the parents themselves truly accept this masculinity and femininity.

The moral component of the child's identity is also highly influenced by his developing sexuality. Immanuel Kant felt that the moral imperative is innate in man. While it is true that rudimentary precursors of a conscience may exist at birth, any parent knows that "good behavior" is neither bestowed by God nor genetic evolution, but must be learned anew in each generation. The child's ideas of good and bad are at first dependent on his desire to please his parents and the fear of their disapproval. His morality, in other words, is not autonomous or transcendental, but is essentially a morality of restraint, of parental control.

The beginnings of an autonomous conscience arise around the fifth year. This development is spurred by the continuing biological maturation of the sexual drive which now becomes more firmly localized in the genital organs and gives rise to a powerful day-dream. To state it in a highly oversimplified way, the core of this day-dream is the young child's sexual and possessive interest in the parent of the opposite sex with corresponding rivalrous feelings toward the parent of the same sex.

Psychoanalysis has called the various components of this day-dream the Oedipus Complex, after Sophocles' tragedy "Oedipus Rex." Under ordinary circumstances, however, this connotation of relentless punishment and inexorable tragedy is only in the child's imagination. Out of the ashes of this tragedy a great advance in the child's sexual and moral development will occur. He renounces the day-dream along with the sexual impulses connected with it. During the period of latency it is gradually relegated to the storehouse of forgotten memories. The energies feeding these urges are freed for use in learning, in play, and mastery of the environment. In its stead there occurs a decisive identification with the parents. The taking in of the qualities of the parents, and especially the parent of the same sex, provides the child with an important stabilizer for his future masculine and feminine mature identity. It establishes as well the foundation for an autonomous moral law within himself.

At the onset of puberty, under the impact of the resurgent sexual drives, the personality integration of latency is disrupted. This reawakening of sexuality in turn threatens to revive the whole gamut of the young persons' emotional interest in their parents, including old and forgotten feelings of dependency and longing. Although the full force of these archaic desires are usually not experienced on a conscious level, the adolescent reacts with various defenses to keep them in check.

Primarily, both the boy and girl attempt to disengage themselves from their parents and to direct these needs to their peers—a direction that is consistent with the demands of healthy development. The urgent necessity for emotional separation from the parents in the direction of greater independence has its long-range rewards, but for the time being it is accompanied by a sense of loss that is reflected in moodiness and a feeling of depression.

This sense of loss that attends the farewell to childhood is similar to that experienced at the end of each decade of one's life: at one's thirtieth, fortieth, fiftieth birthdays, and especially when our children marry and leave our homes, only now—for the young boy and girl —it strikes much deeper, for there is the inner realization that childhood is over and life will never really be the same again. Needless to say, parents, too, find it difficult to separate from their children and to permit

12

them to struggle into a future that leaves their own lives more empty.

The adolescent is caught, in a sense, between the danger of the sexualized and dependent tie to his parents, and the fear of independence and sense of loss that pulls him back to them. In order to give up this supportive relationship of childhood, he must step into the new world of his peers, a world that is devoid of established and secure roles. He must begin to test his abilities, his strength, his fears of the opposite sex, his ideals, and his sense of himself. In doing so he must risk failure and injury to his self-esteem. Thus, rebellion against parents co-exists and alternates with childlike dependency in bewildering succession.

On the one hand the adolescent bristles at the most well-intentioned parental help; on the other hand he will make the most outlandish demands to be catered to and waited on. He will accuse you of nagging when you have to wake him up three times in order to be ready for school. If you wake him only once he will accuse you of not caring whether or not he gets an education. The stronger the dependent need the more violent will be the rebelliousness and anger as a defense against it. I am sure you may be familiar with the experience of parents whose touchy teen-age son is leaving for a date. "Have a good time!" they tell him as he is leaving the house. He answers instantly: "Don't tell me what to do!"

Severe mother-daughter conflicts are not unusual at this stage. They are probably more frequent between mothers and daughters than between sons and either parent. Dependency on mother presents an even greater threat to the girl than to the boy, for it carries with it a threat to the girl's feminine development by intensifying her tie to a woman at a time when she is struggling to achieve a firm sense of her feminine sexuality. For both boy and girl, however, the urgent necessity to relinquish the emotional dependence also means a temporary disengagement from the internalized, psychic model of the parents that has been the foundation of their identity. The rupture of the internalized model results in a fragmentation of the sense of personal identity, which may be experienced as a sense of unreality, a confusion about "who I really am," and a groping for a philosophy of life or an ideology upon which to anchor for the time being a stable feeling of self.

The dissolution of the internalized model of the parents includes as well a partial negation of the values and standards of the parents that have been appropriate to childhood and have served well prior to this time. The temporary negation and realignment of these values is a necessary concomitant to growing up, and to the achievement of an independent and autonomous value system of one's own. Eventually and ideally there will be a remodeling within the personality of a morality based not only on the past, but also on the exercise of judgment and discrimination as applied to the realities and responsibilities of living as an adult in his own generation.

Adolescent sexual attitudes and behavior at first have little similarity to those of a mature relationship between a man and a woman. Sexual feelings as well as the newly-won physical maturity are often felt as alien, and not as integrated components of the self. Frequently the sexual drive is used as an instrument to relieve some of the conflicts of adolescence, for example, as an assertion of masculinity or femininity. With boys there is a great deal of exaggerated boasting with peers about sexual experience. This usually is at considerable variance from the actual facts. For girls it may provide an outlet for defiant self-assertion and hostility to her parents. The adolescent's feelings of loneliness and depression may be temporarily relieved by the illusion of love, created by the physical closeness to another human being. Intimacy with the opposite sex may be avoided altogether because of intense feelings of fear and guilt. Sometimes the negation of the moral code of the parents results in even more rigid self-imposed standards. I am thinking of a young man who, rewarded with a goodnight kiss after a pleasant evening, proceeded to give the girl a lecture about her unladylike behavior!

The sexual behavior of adolescents, as a statement of independence from the parents, is sometimes so extremely specious that only the young people themselves fail to discern it. For example, I would like to cite one young couple, nineteen and twenty-one. During the course of an intense attachment to each other, an illegitimate pregnancy occurred, followed in a few months by a marriage they both wanted. The spurious motive of this sexual independence was betrayed by the fact that both of them proceeded successfully to perpetrate an elaborate hoax on their parents, in which the out-of-wedlock pregnancy was concealed—including the birth of the baby and its placement for adoption—so terrified were they of parental alienation and censure as punishment for the forbidden sexual relationship.

In many instances the guilt over the sexual relationship necessitates idealizing it as love, which may in turn result in marriage. This effects a closure of the adolescent process; a pseudo-resolution that once and for all terminates the search for identity around a premature commitment to a permanent sexual relationship. For an adolescent, it is putting on the cloak of adulthood while carrying into the relationship the unresolved conflicts of the past, and an identity that remains dependent on the childhood image of the parents. Obviously, it is wrong to assume that adolescent sexual behavior and attitudes can be explained only on the basis of a desire for physical pleasure.

Although sexuality can be exploited in the service of more infantile needs, it already has in it the seed of what will become an expression of a deep and intimate bond between a man and a woman. Gradually, near the end of adolescence, these attitudes give way to sexual interest and the need to express it within the framework of a deep emotional bond to a sexual partner. This marks the integration of sexuality into the personality structure, and is an important element in the realization of adult identity.

The harmonious integration of sexuality and morality is influenced not only by the interrelationship of the forces within the personality, but is also dependent upon the social and cultural setting in which these biological and psychological events unfold and reciprocate. At every phase of his life cycle the growing individual meets in his social environment patterned expectations, restrictions, opportunities and an image of himself determined by his society and the particular subculture in which he matures. This social environment can be either positive or negative in meeting the requirements for growth. If it does not meet these requirements, the particular phase of development will run an abortive or deviant course—imposing lasting deformities on the personality.

Since I am limiting my observations to normal adolescent development, I will not deal here with the effects of a pathological environment. I need only comment that the many children raised in slums and ghettos grow up in disorganized families, and are deprived of minimal cultural stimulation. In this setting they develop with a degraded and inferior sense of identity communicated not only by the society that surrounds them, but also by identification with parents whose self-image is already distorted in this direction. They will possess neither the internal stability nor sufficient realistic opportunities to exploit whatever push toward maturity adolescence evokes.

However, for the "average" adolescent in the "average respectable environment" of our society, the acceleration of historical change has produced a wide and ever-increasing gap between the older generation and the younger generation. Within the time-span of a single generation, the march of history has produced unprecedented social, political and technological changes. These phenomena are reflected in such terms as population explosion, sexual revolution, information explosion, and mass communication. There is little doubt that the standard-setting function of tradition has been weakened. In the area of the relationship between the sexes, this is certainly true. The morality of authoritative restraint, enforced by parental control, religious dictum and the economic dependency of women has given way. In the absence of these traditional restraints, the adolescent attempts to resolve his code for sexual behavior within the relationship of his peers. It is possible to assume that the coercive power of these external controls are integrated into the personality in such a way that they then function as autonomous moral directives. While this is true and appropriate in childhood, in adulthood such external controls encourage dependency and inhibit the formation of independent internalized values.

Therefore, if a youth borrows automatically the outward form of another authority, the peer group, little has been gained in moral growth. This fact is behind the fear of the older generation that external standards of sexual license will replace standards of restraint.

The few sociological studies that have been done so far *do* support the existence of a change in the direction of greater sexual freedom among college students. The studies of this rather narrow segment of youth *do not*, however, support the thesis that this change is a revolution in favor of amorality, occasional sensational news articles notwithstanding. They do suggest that the change is in the direction of a more autonomous regulation of sexual behavior which sanctions premarital sexual intercourse within the confines of a serious and exclusive relationship. In only a very small percentage of these studies can the women's sexual behavior be typified as casual or promiscuous. It is highly probable that in these few instances we are observing deviant development wherein pseudo-sexuality is the expression of a serious emotional disturbance, and represents a failure to resolve internal psychic conflicts of adolescence.

18

Observations from another source seem, at first glance, to substantiate an increasing disregard for established social mores. I am referring to the great increase in the number of out-of-wedlock pregnancies; actually an increase of from 10 to 22 per 100 unmarried women over a 15-year period. However, these statistics do not represent a sudden crisis, but a very gradual long-term trend that can be traced back at least thirty years. Interestingly enough, the startling increase is in the age group from twenty to thirty years, not in the teen-age group. The proportion of teen-age unmarried mothers is even slightly lower than in earlier years—in terms of percentages.

Perhaps those who interpret these figures to indicate the breakdown of previous standards and restraints along with the diffusion of a "fun morality" are right. But the evidence is not convincing. Undoubtedly, sociological and cultural changes must be taken into account. From my own frame of reference as a consultant to social agencies working with these young women, the internal psychological causes of the out-of-wedlock pregnancy were striking. For some of them out-of-wedlock pregnancy represented a quasi-solution to an insoluble internal conflict. For others it was an inevitable crisis on the path to adulthood.

The establishment, then, of a firm sense of identity is dependent on the interaction of the various segments of the personality with each other and with the traditions, opportunities, and style of life that the adolescent meets in the world around him. The force of maturing sexuality itself is responsible for the dissolution of the ties to the parents and the shaking up of the whole fabric of the personality configuration of childhood.

In more primitive cultures and more distant historical times, adolescence was curtailed. Under those conditions, the childhood structure of the parent changed very little. The personal identity of the adult was more irrevocably tied to the childhood relationship with the parents, and accordingly, to the traditions, values and standards of the past.

A youth of our society has to weather a more prolonged period of uncertainity and turmoil than any other generation preceding him. He must enter into a new kind of relationship with his peers, where he must embark on a period of experimentation in which he tests his interests and capabilities, his ideals and values, and his emerging sexual identity. Gradually, he will organize into a cohesive whole, with a stable sense of himself that is founded on his unique personal attributes. In this process he is evolving a new kind of sexual morality—a morality no longer dependent for its enforcement on the power of external restraints.

There are the prophets of doom who warn of the disintegration of tradition and morality, and who picture an unsolvable dilemma for the youth of our time. There are the optimists who anticipate that the weakening of the authoritative controls of the past will lead to the evolution of a sexual morality free from irrational fear and guilt, based on independent judgment, reason, and an understanding of adult responsibilities to oneself and to other human beings.

Perhaps it is too soon to tell. I take my stand, however, with the optimists.

social pressures and sexual behavior

WILLIAM DENHAM

■ "When a society is stable and the conditions of life do not change from one generation to the next, though its sex standards may be galling, at least they are clear. When society is in flux, then the emotions connected with the sex impulse itself are complicated by doubts as to what forms of sexual expression are proper and disturbing personal and social conflicts arise between practices and precepts. We are, of course, living in such a time of flux today."

This excerpt from a recent article by Dr. Jerome Frank [1] provides us, I think, with a pertinent starting point. While I might not be able to promise you a new look, as it were, on the topic, it might be useful to look at the social pressure in the context of the era of social change which we and our young people are trying to live through.

Every generation experiences its share of social-cultural strain. However, only certain generations experience the kinds of stress which shake the very fabric of society. We are in such a period. I would like to

Mr. Denham is Assistant Director, Center for Youth and Community Studies, and Associate Professor, Howard University School of Social Work, Washington, D.C.

sketch briefly some of the main social change factors, discuss some of their consequences on the sexual behavior of our youth, and to suggest an alternative which might be considered along with others, in our effort to evolve a more effective system of social ethics.

I would like to discuss four aspects of social change which I believe are of central importance in terms of their influence on sexual mores and behavior: First, the quality and momentum of change; second, the rapid alteration of sexual mores and conduct in youth; third, the bureaucratization of parental functions; fourth, the impact of birth control technology.

Now to the quality and momentum of change.

Seldom in human history have the issues facing society been so survival-oriented and so urgently in need of rational solutions. To mention only a few: The overhanging threat of nuclear war; the population explosion which now threatens to inundate the planet in the foreseeable future if not checked through means other than our traditional recourse to war; the erosion of our natural resources, air, water and land; proliferating demands for educational and training resources to equip our youth with the tools to cope with, let alone conquer, the still only dimly-perceived dimensions of a computerized age; the metropolis going wild in terms of bigness and human and physical decay.

The collective impact of such problems has the effect of undercutting the individual's ability to deal effectively with even one of these problems, such as sexuality. Things seem to get muddled up in our confused, often desperate effort to survive, or, we tend to push away the changes such realities imply.

For example, in relation to sex, rather than recognize

that the sex revolution is irreversible, we continue in many ways to perpetuate beliefs of a pre-contraceptive era in a contraceptive age. Such an ostrich-like response has its parallel in our social policies involving many other crucial issues.

In the international arena, for instance, many of us simply cannot face the reality that the hydrogen bomb has rendered large-scale war obsolete.

Parents and youth are caught up in this multiple impact syndrome. The average parent of teenage kids has not only the youngster's sexual life to worry about, but also his education, the prospect of the draft, and his sociability in peer groups, to mention a few. The youngster, in turn, has to cope with identical pressures, but because he is directly and immediately involved, he cannot work on these problems with the benefit of a perspective.

Self-interest and self-serving strategies are developed by both groups. This is particularly true of communication, an issue which I will return to later. But suffice it to say now, the preoccupation of adults and teenagers with the social problems facing them often encourages the development of isolated systems of communication.

Parents and youth indulge in a process of talking *to* each other. Thus we have what has been termed "the tragedy of American sexuality," namely, the inability of generations to engage in honest dialogue *with* each other.

Now, on the issue of the rapid alteration of sexual mores and conduct in our youth, although statistical indices and expert opinions on the subject of sex may vary, there is general concensus that sexual standards and behavior are rapidly changing. As the excellent report by the Group for the Advancement of Psychiatry titled "Sex and the College Student" indicates, the young are now asserting, with ever-increasing vigor, their right to privacy and choice in their sexual affairs. The double standard is becoming obsolete. Young people appear to be maturing biologically at an earlier age. This report indicates that the average college student tends to go steady earlier, is more articulate in sexual issues, often well-informed about current birth control methods, although, parenthetically, gross misinformation and misunderstanding persist for many, not to mention their familiarity with the abundance of current literature on sex.

The continuing and increasingly intense campus dialogue suggests that students are simultaneously testing authority and looking for directions and functional equivalents for sexual standards which were applicable to other eras, but no longer thought to be sufficient for today.

What is our response as adults? Unfortunately, all too often it has been one of ambivalence or patronization. The "do as I say, not as I do" posture is as archaic as yesterday's Victorian code, and is so perceived by young people.

Or, in some instances, we tend to take the typical stance prevalent in our psychologically conscious era of "counselling" the kid to "adjust or control his impulses." One wonders whether such a response, no matter how well-intentioned, may not be interpreted as Edgar Friedenberg [2] has written as "one of the ploys used by society to disarm the troublemakers among its young—a powerfully institutionalized defense against recognizing that young people might have something valid and

24

realistic to complain about that we can no longer escape from, even when we want to."

How long will we persist in defining misery and discontent in our young people as primarily problems in adjustment? Is this in many instances not a gambit to disarm the agitators? Perhaps we institutionalize the rationale of adjustment so that we are having a difficult time understanding what our young people are trying to say to us.

Now to the bureaucratization of parental functions. Parents are no longer the exclusive source of wisdom and guidance for the young. The role of organizations outside the family, such as the church and school, in supplementing or reinforcing the parental role in the socialization process has been in our culture for generations. More recently, various social welfare agencies, such as family and child welfare organizations, and mental health clinics, have further assumed important functions previously regarded as within the parental bailiwick. As a consequence, parental functions, like other aspects of modern life, have become highly organized—perhaps over-organized. There is no question about the value of these social services which a person in need of help can receive. However, as the demand for help has increased in volume and complexity, services have in turn become increasingly complex and specialized.

Today we find that the human services field is often as cumbersome and complex in structure, purpose and program as the industrial sector of our society. While this may be reality, it still poses a dilemma for youth searching for personal answers to sexual and other problems.

Now a number of questions come to mind. Does the complexity of our social agency system deter many youths, who need a truly personalized or parental touch, from seeking help from this source? Do social agencies tend to promise more than they can really deliver in the kind of personal approach young people look for? Are parents in many instances expecting too much of social agencies, and in the process reducing their roles both quantitatively and qualitatively? "Yes" answers to these questions would call for social agencies and their adult clients to reassess clearly their mutual responsibilities to youth.

On the issue of birth control technology, sexual mores and conduct have come under the impact of rapid scientific change—most dramatically shown in the development of artificial birth control techniques. Authorities tell us they expect a completely effective form of contraception to be available to the general public within a decade. Like so many other scientific advances, the principal question is whether this one will prove beneficial or detrimental to society. Will the "pill" and other devices increase promiscuity and other forms of deviant and emotionally disturbed behavior?

Certainly, we can anticipate that for a minority of young people greater freedom to indulge in sexual intercourse may have negative consequences on the personality. But for a large majority of young people, development in contraceptive technology can provide an opportunity for healthy sexual freedom, depending largely on the capacity of the larger society to make realistic adaptations. Specifically, it will depend on the extent to which the adult world is able to relinquish the elaborate system of myth, mystery and emotionalism which has typified its response to sex over the centuries. This will mean that sex will finally have to be placed within the general context of the whole "style of life"—to use a term coined by Alfred Adler many years ago.

The special role which sex has played in our relationships may need to be downgraded and realigned with other equally if not more vital components of life such as companionship, communication, and the ability to be concerned with others.

Thus far, I have focused on the impact of social forces on the sexual behavior of dominant American middle-class society. The picture, however, would be incomplete without sketching briefly the impact from social pressures on the sexuality of our largest minority, the Negro, particularly deprived and impoverished Negro youth.

Despite the promising beginnings of the anti-poverty program, and the remarkable strides to economic and social equality made by Negroes—in most instances middle-class Negroes—the masses still constitute a subculture or underclass. In mores and behavior this subculture is radically different from the white middle class. This is true in sex and in other areas of life. As many writers have pointed out, the Negro has been denied access into the wider society. Consequently, he has played a relatively minor role in directly influencing the values of the dominant culture.

His response to the social forces I have earlier referred to have tended to be essentially reactive rather than active. His reactions, however, are characterized by a daily grinding struggle to survive in a hostile environment. Life is thus hardened, and prime values are attached to those things which are immediate, available and visceral.

The Negro's sexuality must be viewed in this context, and writers James Baldwin and Claude Brown have depicted this most vividly.

It is fashionable to quote statistics which indicate that the Negro is over-represented in various offical indices of social pathology, including sexual deviation or disturbance. However, these figures do not show us the meaning which lies behind such acts. They do not show us that many poor Negroes attach a primary value to sexual gratification, simply because they don't have any or sufficient alternatives for "making it" in a larger society outside. They do not explain the cavalier attitude of many impoverished Negro boys to the use of contraceptives, nor their promiscuity in relationships.

They do not reveal the real reasons why an unwed mother, herself a product of an out-of-wedlock relationship, is not interested in making even a minimal attempt to find a father for her child. They do not explain the basis of a young mother's fatalistic attitude to the disappearance of her husband. The themes running through such examples can be interpreted as reflecting individual pathology, but such themes more usually reflect the appalling socio-cultural-economic heritage of the Negro.

His two hundred years of slavery followed by almost another century of second-class citizenship has systematically denied him equal social status and the opportunity to obtain it. Thus, it is important to understand that the basis of the Negro male sexuality rests on an unconscious need to impregnate in order to prove his masculinity. However, one might hypothesize that he might never be masculine until he has a real masculine equivalent, such as a steady, adequately paying job, a sense of personal dignity and social power.

Similarly, Negro girls, in their relationships with boys, may continue to act out their denigration of the Negro male until the latter achieves comparable status in a wider society with other men.

What I am saying is that problems of lower-class Negro sexuality cannot be exclusively dealt with in terms of social interventions based on a middle-class morality. Psychological and clinically oriented methods which are used in dealing with such problems should be combined in a therapy package geared to opening up both the psyche and the economic system.

Let me now turn for a moment to the question of birth control as it pertains to the poor. As I said earlier, authorities maintain that simple contraceptive methods will shortly be perfected and made available for large-scale use. We can anticipate rearguard action against their use continuing in various sectors. However, public restrictions are likely to decrease. The present climate of public opinion, therefore, presents social and health agencies with special opportunities to develop programs of sex education for the poor. I would venture that such programs will go a long way toward reducing negative attitudes shared by many poor people about the responsiveness of social agencies to their needs.

Here would be a tangible example of the "reaching out" concept. The importance of well-designed programs should not be underestimated. Programs should be available to individuals and families, and teenagers, on the basis of choice. There is empirical evidence for believing that the poor can be trained to make effective use of birth control information, and thus improve family functioning and reduce unwanted pregnancies.

A recent demonstration involving lower-class Negro mothers impressively demonstrated that short-term group counseling strategies under professional leadership could enable "low-income Negro mothers to control their fertility and function more effectively when exposed to carefully planned professional intervention geared to their value systems and style of life." [3] I would suggest that we might extend this kind of experimentation by training representatives from the poverty subculture as sex educational counselor aides, under the supervision of skilled professionals. In fact, there would seem to be considerable validity for developing intracultural approaches to the highly-charged area of sex education. Throughout the country, evidence is being massed showing that the local professional or semi-professional person can be quite effective in reaching a lower class client.

The New Direction Training Organization, at Howard University, for example, is concerned with the training of dentists' aides and technicians for utilization in health and welfare agencies. And I am always talking about the work of Fred Wiesner at Lincoln Hospital which involves the training of the poor as mental health aides.

If there has been a dominant theme in my comments up to this point, it has concerned the communications gap which exists between youth and adults on the issue of sex, and in many other vital areas of life as well. Social scientists call this the "generations' gap." I would advance two propositions concerning this "great divide." One is that our ability to develop a rational, healthy outlook on sex will be greatly influenced by the extent to which we can bridge this gulf; two, that success in bridging the gap may depend on the extent to which youth can participate in formally influencing the development of more rational standards on issues such as sex, with which they have a mutual concern with adults.

Let us consider two forms of structured group interaction in which youth and adults are really not speaking with one another effectively. First, there are the "policy-oriented" group exchanges, such as forums, conferences, and workshops, which provide opportunity for public dialogue directed to influencing change in community attitudes and standards on issues such as sexuality. Secondly, there are the more "individually-oriented" varieties of group interaction, in which the primary purpose is to meet the educational or social needs of the members. Here are parent education and discussion groups, teenage councils and organized forms of social and recreational activities. Excluded from these categories are the therapeutic groups in which the primary goal is to resolve individual intra-psychic problems of the membership. Also excluded would be the primary types of structured, small groups, such as the family.

One of the major characteristics of these groups is the exclusiveness of membership. Most often they are composed of youth *or* adults, seldom youth *and* adults. Interaction is rarely inter-group. The focus is primarily adult-centered or youth-centered, but seldom adult-and-youth-centered. The issues dealt with, however, such as sexuality, frequently are of equal concern to both. One characteristic common to the youth group is that its agenda and interaction are likely to be controlled or supervised by the adult world rather than by the kids themselves.

This division between youth and adults in group life is especially pertinent to the issue of sexuality. It supports the contention that historically, formal sex standards and practices have largely been defined and promulgated by the adult world.

Youth have been the outsiders, the recipients, rather than the participants. The rationale for this state of affairs has usually been based on the traditional view of youth as immature, ambivalent in terms of their approaching adult responsibilities and overwhelmed by resurgence of their sexual drives and feelings. Less often acknowledged as a key variable, however, is the "hidden agenda" item which concerns the issue of power—the need of the old to maintain their control over the young in respect to their level of maturity, or nature and degree of responsibility which they are directed by their elders to assume. Thus, the power balance between adults and youth is tilted sharply in favor of the adult.

Unfortunately, some of our most progressive organizations—those who are committed to equal rights for young people—often unwittingly exclude them from participation in issues in which they are key actors. For example, should we not have youth participating in this conference? It might have been exceedingly enlightening if, for example, we could have heard youths' side of this subject. We think we know their problem. How would they see the effect of social forces on their sexual mores and behavior? Is this the most crucial question before us?

It is time we began to devise new ways for adapting our group methods to bridging these gaps. One strategy might be for agencies which are committed to improving or changing community standards governing youth conduct to find ways of involving youth in such efforts. The actual participation of youth with adults in various meetings and other forms of public dialogue may prove to be equally as important as any change in values that might evolve.

Another strategy might be focused on the "individually-oriented" group: This would involve experimentation with mixed groups composed of adults and youth, who could be convened to talk about common problems.

On the subject of sex they could discuss a wide range of topics, such as "going steady," premarital intercourse, early marriage, contraceptive practices, abortion, homosexuality.

At first, such groups could be used to bring about a sharing of attitudes and feelings on the subject of sex. Ultimately, they might serve a more basic goal—to move to a more fundamental basis of understanding about their areas of agreement and conflict in all life experiences.

Friedenberg refers to this as the "quest for authenticity." He implies that real dialogue between the generations on issues such as sexual intercourse can lead to social intercourse, in which there is a profound payoff for both worlds. Youth can gain by conveying to adults that in many instances sex is only part of his total view of life. He can also begin to develop a more accurate perception of the older generation. For the adult, the gains would include a clearer perception of the teenage world and his—the adult's—relationship to it; a growing awareness that youth can be allies rather than adversaries or nonparticipants in creating a more sane world.

Finally, I would like to stress that I visualize these types of groups as perhaps being primarily suited for the cross-section of the adult-youth population; the so-called normal population. It is likely that disturbed or alienated individuals could not manage the anxiety and expression of feeling which such exchanges are likely to generate, particularly at the initial stage of confrontation. Even many psychologically sound persons are likely to choose not to go beyond the initial stage. However, the majority will probably elect to do so for the simple reason that, underlying the suspicion, anger or misunderstanding which both groups possess, there is likely to be found the wish to trust, understand and love.

Despite, then, all the *sturm und drang,* there is reason to hope that the present generations' gap can be replaced by a more meaningful and real partnership between the generations.

[1] Frank, Jerome, *The Sex Revolution: New Attitudes on Freedom and Responsibility.* New York: The Ethical Press, American Ethical Union, 1965.
[2] Friedenberg, Edgar Z., "A Polite Encounter Between Generations," *New York Times Magazine,* January 16, 1966.
[3] Russell, M., "A Demonstration Project in Fertility Control." Paper presented at Conference on Parent and Family Life, Children's Bureau HEW, Washington, D.C., September, 1965.

the search for a
meaningful sexual ethic

LESTER A. KIRKENDALL

■ If we are to find a meaningful sex ethic, it seems
to me that three things are necessary. In the first
place, I believe we must develop a more penetrating
concept of what constitutes ethical or moral behavior.
It seems to me that there are several features of the
common concept which need examination. I think that
whenever we speak of morals, and particularly when
we speak of immorality or lack of ethics, we are likely
to think that it's focused in the sexual realm. Actually,
I think that our ethical concepts pervade the warp and
woof of society.

Yet, we talk and act as though it were something
only within the realm of sexuality. We also speak as
though morals were something sort of plastered on, a
poultice, so to speak, or that they are something we
might observe when it suits our convenience. Not long
ago I received a letter from a magazine which was
preparing an article which would feature a series of
comments on the moral situation in the United States.
It dealt altogether with the youth sexual question. They
asked me to pick one from twenty questions and com-

Dr. Kirkendall is Professor of Family Life, Oregon State University, Corvallis, Oregon.

ment on it briefly. As I went over them I found one question which read: "Aside from the possible harmful effects, is it morally right or wrong to engage in premarital intercourse?" So I selected this particular question and started out by saying in essence, well, what is morality? If it is aside from the harm we may do one another, if that is forgotten, then what is it?

I have here an Associated Press story from my newspaper on charting the credibility gap, and it discusses the extent to which government officials lie. I notice that one subcaption here is "Morality Versus Necessity." Again, it suggests that morality is something nice, if it doesn't inconvenience you particularly. For example, it discusses what happened when the U-2 was shot down, when President Eisenhower first denied that there was any such aircraft cruising. The Bay of Pigs is discussed; the three and three-tenths million bribe to the Prime Minister of Singapore. All these exemplify that at the governmental level the use of deception has been very free.

Less than a year ago, we were involved in the Air Force Academy scandal, in which over 100 cadets were expelled for cheating on examinations. In one of the news stories the statement was made that they were expelled for besmirching their own and their country's honor. Now, I submit that in terms of what this story says, these cadets were showing a real aptitude for what was ahead of them. Who can blame youth for being confused? Who can continue to say that the moral problem is a youth problem? Our difficulty is that we have submitted too easily to hypocrisy, to double-talk. This same confusion extends to our sexual realm, of course.

A year or so ago, while the show "That Was The

Week That Was" was still on, I happened to tune in one evening, and heard the commentator speaking about a meeting which I had attended, and they quoted one of the speakers there as saying that he didn't see anything wrong with premarital sexual intercourse, as long as the participants enjoyed it. So, after making this quote, the commentator looked out very intently through the TV screen to the audience and said, "Now, all of you teenagers out there who are not enjoying it, cut it out."

I think that sex has a place for humor. But the thing that concerns me is that we have opened our culture for this kind of amusement and exploitation in which we laugh out of existence standards and principles which I think, along with Dr. Denham, are in many instances outmoded. But we have not yet come to the point where we will do what is necessary to help think through an ethic which will enable us to live in this culture.

One of our problems is to derive our ethical and moral thinking and acting from a basic foundation which is a comprehensive view of what we are as human beings, and what we want out of ourselves and our relationships. I think our concern must rest in a consideration for the quality of relationships which we are able to develop in our families, in our communities, and ultimately, I think, at the international level.

In other words, when a decision or a choice is to be made concerning behavior, I think that the moral decision will be the one which works towards the creation of trust, confidence and integrity in relationships. The decision should increase the capacity of the individual to cooperate, and enhance his sense of self-respect.

This particular point of view was the framework in

which I did the research for my book: "Premarital Intercourse and Interpersonal Relationships, A Basis for Moral Decision-making." And I have found that youth and adults, once they have pushed to the point where they recognize the importance of this approach to themselves and to their families and to their community, begin to search for and accept a very different sexual ethic than we sometimes think they will.

The day is past when we can think of morals and ethics as we did at the turn of the century. Moral concern at that time was centered very largely around the existence of certain vices: drinking, dancing, card-playing, and the major one—sex. The sexual moral code was based on a list of acts which fitted the preconception of a homogeneous community. This code was upheld by stern religious teachings, and imposed deterrents, some of which were at that time quite threatening.

I think this has changed. A meaningful sex ethic must now be derived as a meaningful human ethic. We need an ethical approach which will encompass all human capacities, and which will cut across cultural, ethnic, racial and sex lines, and which will help us survive in the kind of world we have created.

I was interested to note in Dr. Eisenberg's address, and in Mr. Denham's too, that they suggest a part of the moral confusion arises from the intensity of emotions which is part of the collision between the generations. But I have added the concept that our total cultural situation has to be taken into account. As we develop a sexual ethic, it must come through consensus, from interchange, from analysis of sexual experiences and their meanings. Mr. Denham's comments in regard to the place of groups and group interaction were most pertinent. He spoke of the therapeutic type of group. I would extend that, also, to the face-to-face situation in which teachers and youth leaders work with individuals.

I think we must say that we can't change our attitude towards sex and sexuality until it is set in the context of a philosophy of living. I think a different concept of sex is needed. We have, on the one hand, the restrictive, fearful and repressive concept. It is the one which essentially restricts and subdues sexual expression, denies it all through the marriage state, and which defines sexual expression very largely as premarital intercourse.

The second concept, a sort of sex for sex's sake, reflects the fact that when the openness about it developed following the publication of Dr. Kinsey's report, those of us who ought to have been ready with a positive, effective educational approach were not ready. And the mass media moved in with what they had to offer.

These seem to be the extremes of a continuum. The very oppressive and restrictive attitude on the one hand, and the very open and ultra-liberal, if you want to call it that, on the other. Yet, when you begin to examine them, they are very much alike. Both are obsessed with sex as an end in itself. In the one you must not; in the other you must. Both are rigid and demanding, and neither seem really to see or to be concerned with a fulfilled human being.

So I want to suggest the development of a third approach, and this is the one we must work on. I would call it the integration approach; that is, the integration of sex in all of our patterns, because I would like, whenever talking about sexuality, to recognize that it's only one of our capacities. The integration of these capacities into a rich, full, rounded life is the goal. Speaking of sex, there is a time for expression, there is a time for denial, and let us look at both.

Sex is a factor which has significance throughout our lifespan, not simply in youth. I think that one of the important things as teachers is the ability to put sex in a context in which it becomes a part of a touch-embrace relationship. Sexual expression can occur outside this concept, and, of course, this is one of the problems, that it does occur so much outside. But I found that to the young people with whom I work, it has a great deal of meaning to tell them that actually, sexual expression is perhaps an *ultimate* expression, but it isn't an expression of the touch-embrace relationship which we like throughout life.

Whenever we care for someone, parents or child, husband or wife, grandparent-grandchild, male-male, female-female, we like to touch; we like to come close. This is a way of communicating, it's a way of saying something to one another. Yet we have turned sex into such a fearful, isolated, episodic kind of experience that we are no longer able to see it as an integral aspect of this kind of relationship.

We then have to have a new way of looking at sex education. It must be different from the way in which we presently approach it, as something to be told to youth by people who are authorities because they are adults. Now it is something which is imposed from the outside and above, by didactic processes. Study after study, and the experience of individuals, I think, have proved that this is a limited, inadequate concept of sexuality, and not effective, really, in motivating behavior. This does not mean that we should forget reproductive education, the factual information about biology and physiology, but it does mean that we should begin to make a serious effort to look at sex as an integral part of functioning relationships.

We should recognize that sex education is being given to youths who are now in a free choice situation. This, I believe, is one of the major changes that I have seen in my own lifetime. As a high school and college student, I knew friends who broke out of the conventional bounds. But I think that there was much more the feeling of transgression than is now the case. Young people today are open enough, and they are free enough, to recognize that what they will do about sexual participation is a choice which they will make not just once but a number of times.

For example, in a pilot study which I have been doing, I interviewed 131 college men about the choices which they have made: to accept intercourse, to reject it, and to try for it and be rejected by a potential partner, to talk through with a potential partner a pattern which was acceptable to both. I found that on the average, each of these young men listed five and a half such decision-making experiences. Only six out of the 131 had not had this kind of situation with which to contend.

I think that adults often wish it were otherwise, but I regard this as a factor in our culture which will not change. The question is whether we can and will recognize that young people are making these choices, and will we, as individuals, weigh, evaluate, discuss and finally help them get the essential insights which will aid in the decision they make.

One illustration of this attitude I learned at a family

planning clinic in Stockholm, Sweden, last summer. The social worker in charge of the division which was dispensing contraceptive information and devices told me that it was not uncommon for parents to ask for pointers for their adolescent children. Fathers and mothers would come down to the clinic and discuss the questions involved in sexual decision-making. They also had a room to accommodate high school classes which might be scheduled to come to the clinic for the same purpose by their teachers or their principals. She said an interesting thing had occurred a few weeks earlier. A father telephoned to say that his teenage daughter in her late teens, who had been dating a particular boy for some time, had asked his opinion as to whether or not they should have intercourse.

The father was somewhat startled, and didn't know how to answer her. So he asked the social worker for an appointment for his wife, his daughter and himself to discuss the various aspects of the daughter's concern. When the three arrived the social worker was surprised to find the daughter's boy friend had come along, too. Thus, she found herself in a discussion with the parents, their daughter, and the boy friend, on the pros and cons of premarital intercourse, the effectiveness of contraceptives and similar matters.

Few American parents or youth could accept the procedure followed by this Swedish family, but there is an illustration of an effort by a family and a culture to look at the free choice situation.

Audiences who hear this illustration often take it as an expression of the "free love practices" in Scandinavia. I do not see it so. I have visited the Scandinavian countries three times, and while I have little actual research data to support my view, I suspect that we are considerably more irresponsible in sexual behavior than they are in Scandinavia.

In December I drove from Chicago to South Dakota across the state of Illinois. I stopped at a filling station, went into the men's restroom, and found a condom vending machine on the wall. I decided that I would like to see whether this was common practice, so I stopped at several filling stations. In one I really hit the jackpot. This particular station had seven vending machines on the wall supplying a variety of sizes. They had another machine which for a quarter offered pornographic or girlie pictures.

Now, I don't believe that the illustrations which I have just given summarize the whole business; not by any manner of means. I think we have got to come to the point where we teach about this aspect of human living in a total context. The recognition of this need is difficult, and implementing it even more so. It's going to take a very different pattern of thinking than that to which we are accustomed.

The major issue is whether we can honestly and objectively face current realities. The major goal of sex education must be that of helping, with the assistance and cooperation of professional workers in other disciplines, in the development of responsible, mature individuals. We should hope for individuals who will enjoy and be fulfilled by the exercise of their various capacities, including sex, but will exercise them in a context of respect and appreciation of the rights and needs of others.

This is our challenge—can we meet it?

the arts and
the sexual image

Dore Schary

The following comments prior to Mr. Schary's remarks, by Mrs. Barbara Jonas, Chairman of the Conference Planning Committee; Mrs. Sidonie Matsner Gruenberg, Past President of the Child Study Association of America; and Mrs. Herbert W. Haldenstein, President of the Association, help to underscore the changes which have taken place in the approach to sex education in the past fifty years.

CHAIRMAN JONAS: This year we are giving a special award to a very special person, for a book directed to both parents and children. In view of the subject of today's Conference, it seems eminently appropriate to honor one who pioneered half a century ago in what was then the forbidden subject of sex education. Distilled from her long years close to the concern of families and her wisdom, Sidonie Gruenberg wrote a book to be read by parents and children, together or separately, THE WONDERFUL STORY OF HOW YOU WERE BORN. Published fourteen years ago, the book has become a classic. Today, as she completes her eighty-fifth year, we give this special award to Sidonie Matsner Gruenberg and her book.

MRS. SIDONIE GRUENBERG: I am really deeply moved by this tribute. Through my many years of work in this field, several of my books have received medals and such, but to be honored by one's own family, is honor, indeed. Just for a moment, because of my advanced years, I'm allowed to reminisce; I'm not only allowed, but I'm supposed to. And I want to take you, for a moment, to fifty-six years ago, when the first lecture on sex education was given by this organization.

I was then the proud mother of a three-year-old child, and I and other earnest mothers attended this lecture. It was announced as telling your children "the truth." The word sex was never mentioned. This was obviously the only truth we had ever withheld from our children.

So we all knew what it meant.

We were very earnest, and a very nice maiden lady who was steeped in nature lore told us how important it was to tell our children "the truth." And we were advised to go home, think it over and then take a propitious moment, preferably at sunset, to take our child on our laps—our respective laps—and with tongue cleaving to the roof of our mouth, inform them that the stork was not the instrument of fate that he was supposed to be.

This was supposed to enlighten him, smooth his adolescence, and it was very reassuring. And then she also added that the result would be, when we told him this, that the child would throw his arms around his mother's neck and say, "Mother, I love you more than ever now."

So we went home and we tried it. And being child studiers, we were not all surprised at the reaction. Nobody threw any arms around anybody's neck, and they just bombarded us with more and more questions, which we were unprepared to follow through on.

So this was the beginning of it, and I am contrasting it with the meeting today, with all its sophistication, its frank acknowledgement of problems, its social implications, and I think it tells the story in a nutshell of what has happened to Child Study Association of America in every area.

PRESIDENT HALDENSTEIN: Child Study training for professionals goes from Department of Health work to work with adolescents. The objective of one demonstration project, for example, is to equip public school nurses, whose role is also that of guidance counselor, to conduct small, student discussion groups. In them, any subject may be discussed: acne, obesity, personal hygiene, sex, the use of drugs, and, of course, family relationships.

Our most recent experience, which included seventh graders through high school—was really quite startling and overwhelming, and a little frightening. Young people's discussion ranged from old wives' tales and distorted facts of life material to personal experience of the most unbelievable of extremes, including the use of a popular soft drink for contraceptive purposes. The magnitude of the children's need for enlightenment in this area cannot be overemphasized. It is second only to their need for understanding themselves, which is, as we learned earlier from Dr. Morton Eisenberg, basic to their understanding of moral and ethical values of adults. Fortunately, the nurses were well-equipped, not just to answer questions, but to help these young people in their search for self.

Child Study never tries to tell a client—parent or professional worker—how to meet a problem or what to do, but in our training of people for leadership in parent groups, the individual is helped to find his own conclusions. We cannot order another's life, but with understanding and knowledge and skills there are ways in which professional people can be enormously helpful. Today both parents and children are searching for help on the subject of sex education. Their problems in the area of sex do not seem to stem from overpermissiveness on the part of parents, but rather from parental paralysis. Parents want to avoid conflict, but more than that they do not know what to do or what to say.

We believe we must help parents and children search for deeper meanings in regard to sexual behavior and sexual and social ethics. But parents, themselves, must first understand the meaning of adulthood and then be helped to translate this meaning to their children.

For this session we tried to bring you the kind of speaker who brings a well-balanced point of view to our subject. He is not from the academic community, but he holds two doctorates. He is a deeply religious person, but he is not a churchman. He is a leader in organizations promoting civil and minority rights, and in his daily life, in his books and in his plays he demonstrates his awareness and sensitivity and deep understanding of human beings in diverse situations. He is a philosopher who lives and acts dynamically. It is my pleasure to introduce the playwright, Mr. Dore Schary.

MR. DORE SCHARY: As I look at this quite astonishing gathering of educators and professionals, I can't help being reminded of a favorite story of Adlai Stevenson's.

Just before a meeting in Parliament that involved an important issue, Prime Minister Disraeli was approached by a young member of the House who said, "Mr. Prime Minister, do you think I should become involved in the discussion?" And Disraeli said, after a moment, "No, I think it better that people wonder why you didn't speak rather than why you did."

But having a fair sense of responsibility to commitments, I would rather proceed. Stanley Kauffman of *The New York Times,* Walter Kerr of *The Herald Tribune,* and Emily Genauer of the same paper have recently written on the subject of the arts and the sexual image. And, of course, quite depressingly, Hugh Heffner writes incessantly, trying in a valiant way to lift a pleasant enough erotic magazine into a way of life.

However, I think I am expected to dwell on something less obvious; for instance, the nude figure in "Marat/Sade." No; that's fairly obvious and hardly shocking. The second act curtain of "Tiny Alice?" Well, perhaps. In previous speeches and articles I have dealt with these sex images in talking of the theatre, motion-pictures and TV, and the conclusion is inevitable and obviously the same: the arts reflect the society which nurtures and supports it.

I do not argue they should do only that. As a matter of fact, many try to do more but fall as victims before the tidal wave of comedy, music—some of it very good, indeed—and so-called "sick" plays. But if they are "sick" they are symptoms of an epidemic. If we are appalled by some things we see on stage or screen, aren't we just as appalled by the terror of bigots and racists?—or by pollution of the air, water and earth? If nudity is available to the mass public in Kodachrome prints, isn't it a natural consequence that it be available in large screen technicolor, and finally on public display in restaurants, saloons and theatres? If our press is glutted with stories of violence and crime, shouldn't it follow that it be reflected in fiction?

But as we are preoccupied with the need for "entertainment," the subject has to be made palatable and salable, so it follows that sex and violence be glossed over and satirized, and out of this need comes the new school of "camp," which permits us to laugh heartily at copulation and mayhem with no feeling of guilt. Isn't this, too, a reflection, a desire to turn away from the anguished realities?

If your committee intended that their speaker be one who would indict the theatre and all art as the culprit responsible for what appears to be, and indeed is, an escalation of licentiousness and a fracturing of our moral standards, they got the wrong number. The arts are guilty, but so are we. Bad art of any kind—immoral art, irresponsible art—cannot exist without a buying public, and the public is buying. And as the sales increase, the product is applauded for the simple reason that the buyer does not choose to be considered a dolt or a dupe.

"Search for its hidden meaning," my friend says to me, regarding the can of Campbell's soup painted on canvas two feet high. I cannot find any meaning except that an actual can so big could feed a hell of a lot of hungry migrant workers, who would view this present conference as not too related to their unhappy state. They would happily skip a talk on the significance of Le Roi Jones' "The Toilet," for a decent place to sleep.

The truth is that this huge world is a churning, boiling mass of contradictions, paradoxes and predicaments, and art and the sexual image in the arts has little to do with it except provide, in most cases, the tired business-man and his lady with titillation and fun. And if the language is often ribald, catch tomorrow's cocktail party conversation on a tape recorder.

The loose and easy language of social dialogue and of the novel and theatre is designed, we are told, to release us from bondage. The brilliant Kenneth Tynan startled BBC by saying a four-letter word to an audience of millions. Motion-pictures in technicolor and twenty feet tall present for our enjoyment—indeed, our amazement—a bevy of bosoms and buttocks. Seduction is no longer the province of the cad, and we learn that rape is actually something some young ladies look forward to much like a high school diploma.

TV deals with sex as casually as do the other arts, perhaps not as candidly—but don't lose heart—if the competition gets tough enough they'll have to sell soap by selling sexuality. And if violence is so easily and blandly accepted, why not sex? People are killed off in spy stories by the hundreds and it's fun, and no one ever cares. Spear guns pierce throats, knives slit bellies, bullets plow into skulls, knees are thrust into groins, fists smashed into mouths, but no one ever cried—the mass of murdered, tortured, raped, brutalized victims are never buried and never mourned. It takes too long, and no one cares. Insensitized to feeling by excess, the audience only asks, make it more lurid. We are excited, stimulated, amused, and alas, we do not care.

Our attitude about sex is, I fear, in the same state; we no longer care. Sex has gone as public as AT&T. A logical question pops up, and I'm ill-prepared for a definitive answer. I offer only an educated guess as to how we got into this state of crisis.

The awful toll of World War II, amounting to forty-five million deaths, left our feelings paralyzed. How can we feel tne extermination of so many? The death of one person we knew can shock us, but if we tried to absorb in our senses the slaughter of forty-five million, we would go mad; so we build a callous. And as the wars begin again—over forty of them in twenty-one years—yes, forty—count them: Israel, Indonesia, Cyprus, Yemen, Egypt, India, Korea, Hungary, Iran, Iraq, Oman, Malaysia, Vietnam, to name a few—the callous thickens; not all big wars, it is true; not nuclear wars, true; but the ones who died in those small wars are as dead as those in Hiroshima or on Omaha Beach.

Since we are involved in these discussions with sex and family behavior, let's think for a while of our families since World War II. My children, as did your children, grew up in a shadow of conflict. As children in school, you and I were instructed against disaster by fire drills. Our children were drilled and are drilled against the disaster of a nuclear blast; a final, eloquent goodbye might serve them better at such a time. However, they go on being drilled. They are aware of the cold war with its constant threats and the long roll of casualties of the many other wars in strange, far-off places.

The ever-present political climate, haunted by the fear of Communism, is another burr. The burgeoning strength of the Far Right, the missile crisis; all these add to tension. Let us be candid; we have given our children a series of nightmares, some of which remain in their "sub" and "un"-conscious. Our family units have been distorted and often broken. Our children fly to far-off colleges and may travel two thousand miles for a weekend.

In a desperate desire, perhaps born of guilt, our permissiveness has made us afraid to exert parental will. We walk in circles so as not to be called "square," and if our daughters speak quite casually of contraceptive pills, we dare not ask the natural questions that come to mind. Our children, in the main, are a generation of dissenters and protestors. They must look at us and wonder, with some justice, "If your ways are so good, how the devil did we get in this mess?"

We're apprehensive to speak of personal responsibility, because we're not sure that we have performed up to par. We are shy of speaking of morality because we have sinned—or believe we have. We recognize that morality is not a "status quo" of any society. Our generation of the twenties or thirties were to our parents a rather wild group of moral delinquents, and so we are cautious to render a bill of indictment, arguing to ourselves that everything changes, and indeed it does, but to what? Posed against the keystone of behavior of the fifties, which was based on a desire to be "well liked," and we worked hard at that, is an attitude of the sixties: "Who cares?"

Single equations are out, along with God. When we say "Freedom," we are asked what kind of freedom, and for whom? When we say "Peace," we are asked what kind of peace, and for whom, and how do we propose to achieve it? When we say "Democracy," we are asked to define it, and for whom and when?

It is no wonder that so many of our young people

rallied to the civil rights struggle. This was an effort with an end result to be envisioned and achieved. This was something their parents had permitted to endure and which they, the children, would not tolerate. This was an I.O.U. they could pay off and proudly say to us, "What other unfinished business is there around?"

The protest of youth against the Vietnam struggle is not merely a left-wing movement. Of course, there are some Communists involved—but we play ourselves false if we think the motive is purely Communist-inspired. It is, again, the young asking to be heard; asking for new ideas; new constellations of power politics; asking for an abatement of old fears and a recognition of new truths.

If we think they are to be denied, we are totally unlearned. So these young people, as did the Talmud student, rush about, saying, "Ask me a question; I have an answer." They also have questions to which they hear no adequate answers.

I believe then that we, calloused and cautious, are facing a new breed who are eager for new sensations and emboldened by victories. Much of what they say and do we have to encourage; other actions we must be courageous enough to oppose.

We are, of course, intimidated by the guilts and fears which I have already mentioned. Another albatross is our feeling that we are hypocrites. Since we have had, in the past—as Kinsey reported—our own sexual adventures which were handled more covertly, we are embarrassed to address ourselves to overt sex.

Our entire social scheme is based on exposure. We have to know everything. This desire for exposure, in my belief, is reflected in our attitude about sex. Anything and everything goes, just as long as it remains public. Anyone who "views with alarm" is a blue-nosed old fogey of a Puritan. Our dances by rhythm and movement suggest the sexual act, though we might become more concerned if the parties involved stayed closer together One of the delights of the old generation was the act of taking a girl close in your arms and holding her as you danced. Such simple pleasure is as outmoded as the antimacassar.

And this tendency to expose has some positive results. The debates, open and blunt, regarding the War in Vietnam is good exposure. The bustling debates on a score of subjects concerning us is good exposure. What we must guard against is the exposure that is brought upon us under other disguises. As free speech does not entitle us to yell "Fire!" in a crowded theatre, so an open society does not give us a license to embrace a horde of social evils. It is not hypocritical to stand for a code of decent behavior.

The question we ask is, how far and in what direction are we headed? Are we on the path to total moral annihilation, or are we on the path to a new way of life, so free that psychiatrists will have only themselves left for the couches?

There are signs of mortal moral injury. Crimes of youth spatter our front pages, and these crimes do not only spring out of jungle slums. Rich families are tainted by their children who drink too much, smoke "pot," use the "mainline," murder, vandalize, rape and steal. But we hope. We do see signs of health. Colleges are more crowded by industrious and committed students. Theatres and civic centers for music, art and dance are sprouting up all over the country. There are new centers for the humanities. The best of our young people go into the Peace Corps; some to be frustrated, it's true; others to be fulfilled. Young men fight heroically on strange battlefields, even in wars they don't quite understand. Some say there is a revival of religion. The evidence indicates it's a new religion, however, with various rejections of God, but there is a willingness to accept some ethical concepts free of dogma.

So, then, there are three forces working in our society: We, the older generation, puzzled and bunioned; the new "don't care" young men and women; the third is the intense, liberated young men and women who reject some of our old answers to ancient problems, and seek cogent answers of their own. They reject war as a panacea and are horrified by it; they believe in world government; they know what the civil rights struggle all over the world really means; they are generally disamused with Communism and Fascism but seek out new definitions of democracy, and they want to know— as we want to know—where do we go from here?

They have rid themselves of the neurotic tendency to be simply "happy." They want to know about automation and what it means. They do not, in greater numbers than the past, choose to be anti-Catholic, anti-Semitic or anti-Negro. They are not as possessed of ancient fears. If properly supported, they are the champions of the future, but their destinies cannot be determined by clichés and hortatory cant. They prefer the candid admission that we, too, do not know all the answers. A confession of ignorance brings them closer to us as allies in these anxious times. Nothing irritates them so much as the wheezy, "When I was your age. . . ." And indeed it is a wheeze, for the plain truth is that "when I was a boy" has very little to do with when my son was a boy.

I grew up in an age of illusion. Banners waved and drums rolled and we walked along with the doughboys as they set off to lick the Kaiser. Cowboys were all heroes, Indians were all villains. It was a simple age when we believed that the Emancipation Proclamation, way back in 1863, had solved everything for the Negro; when every world crisis could be handled by a regiment of United States Marines; when it was clear that Europe and Asia were too far away for us to be alarmed by empty threats.

In that time, planes which could carry twenty people were speculations on the cover of *Popular Mechanics*, and radio, television, satellites and space vehicles were as visionary as unemployment insurance, Medicare and old age pensions.

So the "when" of today is what we have to contend with. Weary as we are, we have to renew our energies. Calloused, we have to rub our skin free and be prepared to be hurt and sensitive. Otherwise, we will miss what our young people are trying to say. I would hazard a guess. They want us to stop being so permissive to them; to everything. They want us to join with them in fashioning fresh affirmations of faith. They want some deep and righteous—not self-righteous—moral indignation.

I believe that in this widespread preoccupation with sex and violence we are forgetting to be indignant about the horrible intransigency of some of our Southern politicians, or of the stultifying influence of ninety percent of our television programs, or of the overwhelming drive that is forcing us into obnoxious conformity, or of the shifting values that have substituted status symbols for lofy ambition, or of our deteriorating position in world affairs, or of the helpless and almost prone position of our teachers, or of all our commercials that assure us that life is sublime if only we smell sweet, have white teeth, use soft tissue and smoke a cigarette that is tar-free.

How can we carp at our children if they know papa and mamma get fairly well stoned at the Country Club, and that papa foxed the Internal Revenue Service out of a fat check by phoney expense accounts?

This breakdown within the family cuts across all class lines. The slum families provide little incentive by coming home drunk from the corner bar or by proudly setting a stolen transistor radio on the table. Public and private schools bear scars of a tormented family structure, and what is required is a clear-eyed recognition of the unpleasant truth, and then a determination to do something about the situation.

What I am urging is a whole-hearted attempt at individual responsibility in every activity of our lives. As with bad art, we cannot legislate bad behavior out of our lives, nor wish it or talk it out of existence. We can only act it "out" by personal behavior.

There is a joke about two ladies discussing vacation plans. One lady says she has no idea where to go; she's been everywhere. The other lady asks where the first lady went last year. She answers, "I went to Aruba." "Where's that?" she's asked, and she answers, "I don't know; we flew."

As with all jokes, there is truth to behold. I submit that we today know we have gone some place and how we got there, but we haven't the foggiest idea where we are. And if we don't, how do we expect our young people to know? I think together we can find out. It means stripping away caution, fear, worn-out custom and new-fangled permissiveness. Tolstoy said that all of us want to change humanity, but we are not willing to change ourselves. Well, let's change ourselves. We might be amazed at the fine reception we get from some of our kids, and how eagerly they will change with us. Art will also change because its mirror will catch a different reflection.

But the arts and the people who work in it have individual responsibility beyond their own enclave of endeavor. They are the communicators—in theatre, films, TV—the written word and the painted form. They have to move out of their ivory towers and smoke-filled pads and do something beyond just reporting what goes on. They could and should blow the whistle, ring the alarm, sound the tocsin, and wake up the people. They have—along with us—to learn to care; care hard.

Carlyle said that man forever stands at a door; if he fails to open it he is doomed to say on his fours and root in the mire as a beast—if he opens the door he will walk straight and tall. We are still at the door. Let's open it and walk into a new world.

the issues for parents

AFTERNOON PANEL DISCUSSION

CHAIRMAN,
MRS. MILDRED R. RABINOW

ALGERNON D. BLACK
MARY S. CALDERONE
SAUL SCHEIDLINGER
HELEN F. SOUTHARD

CHAIRMAN MILDRED R. RABINOW: We have invited
as members of our panel four who represent different
professional groups. On my left is Dr. Mary S. Calderone, a physician and now the Executive Director of
SIECUS, Sex Information and Education Council of
the United States, Inc.

Mrs. Helen F. Southard represents the psychological
profession. She is a psychologist who is Associate Director of the Bureau of Research and Program Resources of the National Board, YWCA.

Dr. Algernon D. Black, a religious leader of prom-
inence, and now a senior leader of the New York
Society for Ethical Culture, is also the author of a new
book for children, THE FIRST BOOK OF ETHICS.

On my extreme right we have both the social work
and the psychology profession represented by Dr. Saul
Scheidlinger, who is Group Process Consultant of the

61

Community Service Society, and Associate Clinical Professor of Psychology at the Albert Einstein College of Medicine, New York City.

Our panel members have had experience working not only with a limited class population, but with young people as well who come from different class structures in various parts of the United States.

We have asked the panelists to give a short presentation based on the dilemmas that parents and young people have brought to them, as well as what they consider to be the critical parental concerns of various groups in our population. We will start, first of all, with a gentleman who claims that he really doesn't have any answers, that he is here only to ask questions: Algernon Black.

DR. ALGERNON D. BLACK: This really shows that there is very little ethics in the world because this was unplanned. And the Chairman clearly has no ethics whatever, for I was supposed to be the last speaker!

One of my questions is the relation between morality and ethics. I suppose philosophers would differ and theologians would differ, but I have one way of looking at it which I will express for myself. That is, every culture has its moral code, and the child is brought up to believe that certain things are right and wrong or good and evil; that this is the accepted way to behave, and this is what is expected of people, and that is the morality of that culture, whatever it may be.

As anthropology has uncovered the great variety of cultures, so has it uncovered the great variety of moral codes. And so, in history we see the changes of moral codes. If a person violates the moral code, doesn't live up to it, we consider him immoral, I suppose, in that society context.

But suppose he passes a judgment on the code. Suppose he says, "This is not moral," or "This is not good." He presumes to make his own value judgment. I think, when I use the word "ethics" I refer to the individual making a judgment on the moral code. For example, the moral code of slavery—which in a narrow sense dictates that the slaves should obey the master, take care of him, serve and be loyal, and that the master should take care of the slaves—doesn't necessarily question slavery itself.

At a certain point people begin to talk about or make an ethical judgment on the morality of slavery. And so we get abolition. We get emancipation. We move to a society in which we say, "No one shall own anyone else."

The same would apply in the area of sexual relationships. At a certain time it is accepted as moral that one should not mention this subject in polite society, nor expose parts of the body, nor express oneself in public beyond a certain point, nor lose one's virginity, nor discuss or teach birth control. All these things could be considered immoral, and immoral people do these things, and they violate the code.

Yet, the people who have violated the code in these many cases have not done it out of selfish ego or disregard of other people, but because they cared so much about a more ethical society.

And so we are today wrestling with what *is* the ethical judgment on the moral code of sex in American culture today?

We are living in America in a pluralistic society;

many influences have broken up what formerly seemed to be a fairly set code. Some of the influences from other countries and from other cultures have challenged our ways. But also it comes from within the culture because the code is no longer realistic. It is no longer possible to live by a code which is outmoded.

In a pluralistic society one cannot simply bring up people to accept a given moral code; more than ever, it is urgent that we face the diversity of moral attitudes and practices to help our children find a way of directing themselves. It is not then any longer a question of imposing a moral code, but of preparing people for the responsibilities of freedom.

I think that parents instilling values in children by which they can make their own decisions and their own judgments is something that has to begin very early. It may not be so much a matter of talking and teaching as of the whole climate in the home of respect for persons, and the level and quality of relations among the family. In this context, frankness and even projecting ideals of life could take place with some integrity.

DR. MARY S. CALDERONE: My experience, first as Medical Director of the Planned Parenthood Federation of America and now at SIECUS, has principally been with college and high school students in suburban or small-town areas of middle and lower-income levels.

If we are to change set attitudes about human sexuality, I believe that this middle group is the group to try to reach first, not only because of its numerical preponderance, but because it is in this group that one can see the phenomenon of wanting to do something to make things better in society. However, once we prove to young people that we not only want to but can talk with them about sex in a non-judgmental and objective fashion, then socio-economic levels will be no bar. One girl said in a magnificent interchange between adolescents, "The trouble with grownups is when they want to give us sex education, they don't want to educate us, they just want to control our morals."

This is true, profoundly true.

With regard to the sexual behavior of their children, I find most parents fear and are concerned about the wrong things. They don't want their daughters to get pregnant nor their sons to get involved.

It would be more constructive if they directed their concern earlier to the chain of events that lead to such undesired eventualities. But if they do so at all, it is usually in terms of the looks of things rather than in terms of the ability or inability of their children to relate to other people in creative and constructive ways, and to make intelligent, responsible decisions in all aspects of their lives, which would of course include the sexual.

It is time that adults began to be aware of certain important factors in our efforts to understand human sexual behavior under present societal conditions. They are changing very rapidly.

First is our tendency to equate sex with coitus. This narrow and rigid concept has succeeded in focusing our young people on the genital and erotic aspects of sex. Second is our identification of coitus as a thing to be exploited, so that a thing-centered society then uses sex as a thing, and the people use each other as things. Third is our inability to recognize and accept the valid and indeed the essential sexuality of all ages from birth upwards to the end of life. This is particularly true of parents in regard to their adolescents. There may be seeming acceptance by the parents that their children are sexual beings, but only in terms of the externals, the trappings of femininity and masculinity. Fourth is our confusion of morality with moralisms, with these latter quite properly rejected as non-pertinent by our young people.

But we do not balance it by making clear in our schools and churches that these moralities, Mr. Black, are those by which human beings must live all the same. They have to be the same for all relationships, whether interracial, interreligious, international, inter-social or interpersonal, including sexual. This is why you can and must teach the moralities in the schools, and religion does not have to obfuscate this issue. The old moralisms are always couched in negative terms—things we should not do. But moralities can be worded positively in terms of things we can, should want to, and must do.

Fifth is our inability to admit to our young people that sex is marvelous, creative, varied, and a colorful experience, and fun and funny, incidentally. But this is so rare when sex is limited to the genital level or when it is claimed as a right, before emotional maturity has earned it as a privilege.

What guidelines then can parents give? At this stage in our rapidly changing society, I would tell you that I don't think parents are the best people to give sex education—not reproductive information—but sex education to their kids because it imposes too great a burden on the parent-child relationship at a moment when it is most stressed.

Some of the questions we are asked tell us that. The kids ask us, "Where can we go to get our questions answered and our anxieties talked out? We can't go to our parents because right away they say, 'What do you want to know for?'"

I have a last suggestion. We don't accord to our young people the respect and the attention that they are entirely capable of commanding. If we did, we would need only to go to them and open the discussion. We level with them. They level with us. We have to begin the dialogue and keep it open if we are to ever resolve all of the many difficulties that we now see in this area of man's being.

In view of the explosive dangers we now recognize when the talents and energies of adolescents are bottled up and given little constructive outlet in the running of society, I would urge that young people of all classes be involved in such projects as Headstart and day nurseries. Awareness of how the young human being can be helped to develop into a whole man or a whole woman is as essential a part of reproductive biology and sex education as any other; perhaps more so.

The youngsters I meet know that something has been wrong or missing in their own nurture. In helping small children overcome these lacks, they will find, I believe, some of the rectification and healing that we must make sure they get.

DR. SAUL SCHEIDLINGER: Ten years ago when I left the comfortable field of applying group processes with middle-class populations, and began to work in the education and treatment of the socially disadvantaged,

I learned that I am not really an expert. A kind of identity crisis occurred. And so, like Dr. Black, I will be engaging in a dialogue, but not offering really full final answers, because my colleagues and I are still involved in challenge, concern, and trying our models.

Before we can speak about the concerns of parents in the poor neighborhoods of a large city, one must keep in mind the social climate of the neighborhood, and the unique problems faced by everyone living or working there.

To begin with, there are the unmet physical needs —extremely low income, larger-than-average families with inadequate housing, poor health, overcrowded schools with insufficient medical and social services. Hand in hand with these goes the less-talked-about but even more devastating psychological factor of discrimination, with its humiliation and lack of opportunities for advancement which is part of the minority group status.

Professor Denham mentioned some of these elements. And yet, despite the dire physical and psychological needs, despite the higher delinquency rate, the larger numbers of addicts, of prostitutes, of disorganized families and illegitimate births, the concerns of most of the parents are not basically different from those encountered in so-called middle-class neighborhoods. They too are concerned about what companions their children have, about their use of leisure time, about issues of discipline and control and, above all, about the impact of the environment, of the public media which Mr. Schary talked about, and of the street morality on sexual attitudes and behavior.

What are some of the elements in this street morality to which youths in so-called ghetto neighborhoods are frequently exposed? To begin with, there is the adage, "All things are better if they are fun." Considerations of mature values and regard for others give way to an emphasis on momentary excitement and gratification. Apart from the double standard regarding sexual behavior, there is the notion that manliness is expressed through aggression, never through emotional closeness. In this street morality, the relations between the sexes are devoid of any give and take, with males and females being temptations and threats to one another.

In the face of these factors, it is not surprising that some parents who have families in which there is steady employment, stability and religious morality, in their anxiety, go to the extreme of becoming overly traditional, authoritarian, and even more puritanical than middle-class parents. The ensuing threats and coercion often deepen the gap between themselves and their teen-age children.

A smaller group of families in the disadvantaged neighborhoods have become weakened by the frequent personal pathology and by the repeated crises and pressures of daily living to the point of disorganization. These are likely to be large households headed by women who derive their financial support from public welfare. Apart from the inadequate way in which physical needs are met in these homes, there are the problems of the absence of a reliable successful model of a father, who besides being a breadwinner can be a symbol of authority, protection and a source of moral standards. (I would not like to imply that these roles are being filled by middle-class fathers without complications and conflicts.) Many of these mothers are so overwhelmed by the necessities and demands of their daily lives and by tending to the needs of their younger children, that their influence and control over their teen-agers is tenuous and usually non-existent.

It is with these families that society's care-taking institutions—the school, the church, the public and private agencies—face the greatest challenge. Here material support and psycho-social guidance is essential for the parents, as well as for the children, for in the face of current realities, neither can do it alone.

While I have stressed the unique nature of the physical and social realities which color the sexual concerns of parents in a socially disadvantaged area, it must be remembered that the similarity in basic concerns of all parents, regardless of cultural or economic status, by far outweighs the differences.

There is not a single social problem or distorted value in today's urban ghettos that is not present to some extent in the most advantaged neighborhoods, for people's fundamental needs and the complex forces of modern society are basically the same for all.

MRS. HELEN F. SOUTHARD: I consider it a great privilege to be able to meet with as many groups as I do—groups of young people, yes, very young,—seventh, eighth, and ninth graders on up through high school and college. I also meet with the parents of these young people in small groups, small enough in each instance to allow people to express their deep fears and convictions. On some occasions I have had young people in with the adults, and this has brought forth some interesting responses which I will speak of in a moment.

I meet, too, with you leaders. I feel very deeply

about all the people with whom I work, and the more I work with them, the more I am unwilling to draw generalizations, because I realize how much each person, parent, leader, or youth is a product of his own upbringing, each with a different outlook on life. But I am going to venture a few generalizations, for I think that many of us get so used to talking about this subject that we tend to overlook the terrific trauma many parents have when they hear the things young people are saying and thinking.

I find many parents who believe that it is other people's children who are in trouble and not their own. Often when I will be talking with a mother, and she will say, "I am so glad my daughter could be here at this talk. I don't have to worry about my own children, but I do think it was important," a youth leader will later come to me and say, "You know, that woman you were talking to, you may not know it, but her daughter is in deep trouble." I think this is something that we have to remember, as leaders, and realize that the idea of their children going off the rails shakes parents to the roots.

Many parents are concerned more about the ultimate happiness of their children than they are about sexual difficulties that might arise along the way. Mothers of daughters will say that they really want them to be popular and not to be considered out of the group. They want them to meet enough interesting people to find a marriage partner and have a happy life. This is what is uppermost in their minds. This is the thing that causes the pressure. This is what causes the young people to feel that they must conform to the group.

Still mothers have great ideals for their children.

Many mothers of young boys have said to me, "I wish the girls wouldn't be so aggressive and call them. I am so afraid my son will get trapped into a premature marriage before he has been able to go on and finish his education." I hear this worry just as much as I do that she might get pregnant or that he might get her pregnant.

Sometimes of course when I have had young people in the group with parents, I find that this parental trauma can be more easily accepted. But on one occasion when a group of college students were speaking about the situation today and saying, "Well, after all, there is no right or wrong, whatever you think is right is all right, and it is up to you to make the decision," the mothers came to me and the adult leaders afterwards and said, "You must have put ideas in these girls' minds. They didn't really say that. They couldn't have said that unless you had influenced them."

This is not an isolated incident. To me it is indicative of something that as leaders and as parents we must grapple with.

I think it is much easier for us to deal in the abstract with some of these principles than to bring them down to reality and implement them. When I am with a group of leaders, they say, "All right, now what do I do when my client comes to me and says, 'What contraceptives can I use?'" Or when a girl comes and says something about her relationship to her parents. It is really very difficult sometimes to have the answer. We professionals often talk about the needs of the whole individual or perhaps we call it "the developmental tasks." We know full well that it is very important for everybody to learn how to love and to be loved. We

72

learn how important it is to break the ties of dependency and to become independent persons. We know how important it is to have a good self-image, to feel positive about one's self, to know what it means to be a man or to be a woman. We know how important it is to have some kind of values.

We can say these things and we have been saying them, but now let me translate some of them into the problems of today and see whether we are doing all that we can do to help our young people make responsible decisions.

When it comes to breaking the ties of dependency, the concept is fine. But when young girls go out with a group for the first time and the guys go off to a motel, and some of the sophisticated girls are expecting to have sexual relations, and some of the seventh, eighth and ninth graders are not prepared for it, then they must make a decision as to what they will do. Has anybody talked with them about independence and what this means when you bring it down to this kind of breaking parental ties?

We don't know what it means to be a woman today. I don't think we have really explored the new dimensions of womanhood in 1966, where woman has within her own hands for the most part the choice of whether or not she is going to have a child, the opportunity to be aggressive about dating, and to be extremely aggressive in the relationship—which was not woman's role at the turn of the century.

Some of the new dimensions of manhood, if we had time, we could go into. But that would bring up the whole question of what it means to be a man today dealing with a woman such as I have described.

When it comes to values, it is very easy to talk about being a good girl or good boy. But when it comes to the intellectual exercise of going over all the values that one has, throwing some out and keeping certain ones, when this happens at too early an age, this is threatening. It is all right to do this when in college, but it is a little hard to take when one is in the eighth grade.

The last point in relation to the developmental tasks that I want to mention is the one about getting information. This may sound trite, but we have said to children over the years, "Learn all you can. Go out. When you are in kindergarten, go to the firehouse, go to the dairy, ask all the questions you want."

But now when the child gets a little bit older and asks questions such as we are asked in our groups, this is different. An eighth-grader will ask of the leader, "What does sexual intercourse really feel like anyway?" Some people are not prepared to answer it, and that is the understatement of the year.

But ultimately, I am very hopeful that this is the time for those of us who believe in the strengths and wisdom from our rich Judeo-Christian heritage to sift them out and be vocal about them.

DR. BLACK: Instead of going in a wide range of questions and discussions, I wish we could block this down a bit. I wonder if we could stay a little while with sex education first—though I know that is not a narrow subject—but I meant in terms of how and where it should be started.

We know that in many homes the parents are unable to deal with even the facts of where babies come from or the biological material. The school is one place where this could begin, and I suppose part of the problem in America is that most of the schools don't do anything about it. The parents for the most part in this country assume that politics and religion will be handled in the home, and religion in the church and temple besides. But most parents don't expect the school to do anything about sex education, and many of them would not want the school to do anything about it. This is one hurdle that I think we would have to overcome.

Part of the hurdle is that parents have a problem themselves—maybe we all do—in understanding what it is, maybe more than the children have. If you are a teacher in a school and offer to teach the course, the principal will very often say, "Well, that is up to the doctor and the nurse. Those are the people that know how to teach this. We don't want anybody else to touch it." That means they are calling for scientifically factual material. Or he may say that the biology teacher should do something about this. They all might even be wise enough to realize that this information should come at different stages; that is, there is the pre-puberty stage of fifth and sixth grades, then the puberty stage of junior high school age. Then it may come in a different form for the older teen-agers.

When we at the Ethical Culture Schools come to the sexual question in the ethics classes, so-called, it is considered part of the larger study of human relations. In those sessions there is a give and take. If there is an atmosphere of trust, of people sharing experiences and asking questions and exchanging views, then this could be a very healthy atmosphere.

Most public schools don't have a plan for this. I

suppose some have life adjustment problems or life problems or human relations sessions in which they try more consciously to bring about a reflection of the implications of our behaviors, parent-child relations, attitudes towards money, politics, the race question, and the whole area of human relations.

I would like to give an example of one technique that we have used in our schools. We have asked children to submit, without necessarily signing their names, two or three questions that they consider are basic in such areas as: my attitude toward myself, toward my home and family, in relation to the school, in relation to community problems, and even finally toward death. Selected questions in the family area are then dealt with in the classes.

I should like to ask this as one of my many questions: do you go along with this approach to the beginning of the building of sex education in the schools as part of the human relations program?

Of course, in every class there are children who are precocious, or more sophisticated, and children who are maladjusted or exhibitionistic. I am speaking now as a teacher with experience, who has some sensitivity to the fact that all are individuals at different stages of development, mental and emotional.

There are also children who have certain sexual experiences very early and have blockages. You can do excellent sex information work, but that child may not get a thing out of it personally and will just let the curtain down on it.

With classes of those in the teen-age years, one of the interesting facets of the many discussions on sex education are the answers given to: when did you first learn about this and how and where and from whom? One of the things that comes out is that they wish parents would begin earlier to teach them whatever they can, and, second, that they wouldn't be so gun-shy.

But they come to the conclusion that they are not sure parents should do it because parents have "a bias." If you probe that and say, "What do you mean by a bias?", they will say, "Well, they are conservative; they are old-fashioned. They don't know or they won't answer honestly or their ideas aren't relevant, aren't realistic."

Then you say, "What makes you think they are conservative? Is there a reason?"

They answer, "They are over-protective. They are afraid for us. That is why we can't trust them to answer our questions as we can some other person."

In my senior classes at the high school, I write on the blackboard three propositions. Some of you may feel these are pretty shocking. I will tell them to you because although they seem perfectly okay to me and the students I deal with, I don't know whether you could do this in the public high schools with the seniors.

The first proposition I will put on the board is this: The parents of this school believe that their sons and daughters should not have sexual intercourse before marriage.

The second proposition is that the parents of this school do not believe that their sons and daughters should ever be in a situation where they could be seduced, raped or express themselves sexually and affectionately to the point of "no return." That is delicately put, I think.

The third proposition is that the parents of this

school do not know what their sons and daughters think about this or do about it.

Then I will say to the class, "Are these propositions true?" From this flows quite a discussion. This is a group of intelligent students who have a great deal of information by this time. They have gotten it from everywhere, including the mass media, talk, discussion, and reading. Out of our discussion come specific questions which they want answered.

But how much can sex education in other schools include the kind of approach I have suggested? I am asking particularly for Dr. Calderone to answer some of the questions I have put.

DR. CALDERONE: As usual, I have no pat answers because we are feeling our way obviously. Everybody is. Helen Southard and the Y.W.C.A., however, have prepared some magnificent materials in record and pamphlet form that can form the baseline for what I always recommend to every community:

No teacher, no doctor, no nurse, no one person in the school should say, "These kids have got to have sex education and so I am going to do it." I do believe that until we know more of what we want and what we need and how to go about it, that what a community gets in the way of sex education should be what the community wants, and has planned for.

The program may be very limited in our minds, but if it is what the community wants, it will mean that doors are not slammed and that some progress and change will be made. I think this is very important.

Certainly all of these detailed decisions whether boys and girls meet separately or together, and when and at what age do you say what—I think all of these will fall into place after we first feel our way and plan to do what we know as a community we want done.

Some parents, clergymen and I have just taken part in a community program marvelously prepared in the state of Washington, in which I was sponsored by the Medical Society Women's Auxiliary, the ministers, the Y.M.C.A., and the college. There were a total of six or seven community organizations that sponsored my being there and had prepared for four months before my coming.

All I did was come and speak to ten groups, including young people, in 36 hours. They had done all the ground work and were ready to go. All I did was give them courage to take the final step on their own. (There are, by the way, syllabuses and there are curricula available which are listed in one of our SIECUS newsletters.)

So the most important thing is for the whole community to become involved. Eventually the whole school should be involved—not only the biology teacher and social sciences and family life education teachers, but the English teacher in discussing "The Scarlet Letter" will not be afraid to discuss the basic theme. How was adultery looked upon in that particular time? How was it treated? How do we treat it today?

I think that we ought to be throwing out to the kids many questions. For instance, what is marriage for? Let them debate why is marriage still a much sought for phenomenon in our society. What is sex for besides reproduction? Who makes the pre-marital decisions? This is a red-hot one. It has to do with the relationship, which is a changing one, between men and women.

The girls resent having to be the one to say "No" or the boys push and see how far they can go. The girls are wondering why, at all ages, the boys shouldn't share in making the decision; and they feel that the old argument that it is the girl who can have the baby and therefore she should say no has nothing to do with it.

The high school is our last chance to rectify many of the gaps that exist because of what we have not done, and we have to involve the kids themselves. Sometimes the men want to ask questions alone, such as what does orgasm in a woman really feel like? What does it do? Or, "What do men really do when they have a homosexual relationship? How do they do it?"

I have come to realize that many boys have homosexual advances almost inevitably made to them, and it has never been explained to them that this does not mean they themselves are potential homosexuals. Many of them go off their schoolwork and almost have breakdowns because nobody has explained this.

I never worry about the unsuitability of questions, for I have seen groups deal with them beautifully. The boy who goes too far out on a limb or says something off-color is immediately sat on by his friends—once they respect you because you respect them.

And finally, they ask about this business of the point of no return. What do we mean by the "point of no return?" Do we mean that a penis has entered a vagina? That is why the Swedes think we are immoral, because by our silence we countenance total sexual intimacy in every orifice of the body to mutual orgasm provided the penis hasn't entered the vagina. They consider that hypocrisy.

CHAIRMAN RABINOW: I think that Dr. Calderone is showing why so many people feel frightened about trying to handle some of these questions because it takes courage to answer them. I know that whenever I have done sex education work with adolescents, they ask all of them. You really must be prepared and know that if you open the door they will ask them.

DR. SCHEIDLINGER: I would like to comment on the remarks of both Dr. Black and Dr. Calderone from the point of view of someone who is interested particularly in using the small group for these purposes.

The adage that the beginning worker in this field is told to start where the group is—is the group ready— will answer in part the concerns that Dr. Black expressed. You start where the group is, but the next question here is: Is the leader ready?

I think it is preposterous at this point to ask, for instance, that the public school system conduct sex education, because there are many teachers who, if you asked them, wouldn't want to do it. I don't think any teacher should conduct sex discussions with her groups unless she wants to, and, if she wants to, unless she gets some help in how to do it.

In other words, I am not concerned so much about little models or techniques, whether one leader will be more comfortable in talking to girls alone and another with boys and girls. The question is really one of attitude. As you even hear some of the people here at the table, you realize it is their attitudes that do the job of educating. Young people today want a sense of commitment, leadership, values. The apathy that leaders so often complain about among young people is there because the leadership does not provide a commitment. Just look at what happened in some of the southern cities when leaders did show a way to very apathetic and very deprived people. They moved with them.

I think those are some of the considerations to keep in mind when we talk of mass educational programs in this sphere.

MRS. SOUTHARD: I think while it is true that leadership is important and there is a leadership question, I think leaders can grow in their ability not to be thrown by the subject.

I have known people who after sitting in on three and four sessions have said, "Well, I feel more comfortable. I don't know all the answers, but I am not quite so shocked by it now."

This is why I believe that we all can begin to do bits and pieces. The whole program doesn't have to be done at once. I think a school—that is, the PTA, or even some other organizations, such as Y.W.C.A.—could work with mothers of kindergarteners. There could be some pilot projects where one could experiment with discussions of literature.

But I am convinced that there is a whole new healthy climate. There is waiting a great deal of support from people in the community, and I think there are things many of us can do which will strengthen the persons willing to undertake the teaching.

And I am all for leadership training to get courage and insight, even though not all of the professional answers will come across at once.

CHAIRMAN RABINOW: I wonder if for a moment we can get back to the dilemmas that occur in families where perhaps there are parents who would go along with many of the concepts that we have talked about, but are faced with problems they can't quite answer.

One of the questions, for instance, from our audience was: "As a parent of a freshman college student, I have had a number of talks with our daughter on sex relations. I find she plans to experience sex as part of a living experience and does not think it unethical or wrong. Frankly I do not know how to cope with this attitude."

Apropos of this, I think many of you have read an article in a 1966 issue of *McCall's Magazine* that reflects some of this concern about "What do the parents of a young adult do about the kind of questions they are confronted with?"

There is one statement in this article from a mother which I would like the panel to react to: "Because as her mother I am in a very special position, everything that I say is fraught. It is nonsense to believe I am just another opinion in a world of many opinions. Her father and I are the givers and takers away of approval and permission. Ours is the sanction like no other. We are conscience, and that I think is how it should be."

DR. BLACK: One of the interesting things to ask teen-agers is, "How is the sexual experience different from eating and drinking? They are both physical acts."

You don't need to spell out to them the delicacy of the emotional and aesthetic feeling, the concept of coming close to someone, of a fulfillment, of a sense of the beauty and meaning of life. Nor do you have to spell out for them that when you start to bring a life into the world, this is a responsibility. They know that.

But I am talking about young people who haven't been coarsened, or in whom sex hasn't been separated from the emotion.

I think that in offering sex education there should be respect for the sensitivities and the tenderness and the emotion and the romantic feeling, as well as the attempt to inform and be frank about it. But there is no great virtue in frankness where you drag everything out into the open. There are ways of saying things. They know perfectly well what you mean without necessarily talking about the penis and the vagina.

I don't go with Dr. Calderone at all, that it is any virtue for adults who have suddenly become emancipated to trot this out on sensitive kids in adolescence. I think that you could, without thought, really destroy something in children. I am speaking about a group learning situation now, not about an individual sitting down with you alone. That is something else again.

But I believe that when we undertake this, those of us who undertake it need to give some kind of assurance that we will not just be talking about meat.

CHAIRMAN RABINOW: In fairness to the article that I referred to earlier, this mother makes the distinction that you may go on saying to your children how you feel about relationships, about love, about marriage, about life, but you cannot insist on invading their privacy.

Dr. Calderone was speaking before about the attitude young people have when you are talking to them: they suspect you are really out to investigate what was their last sexual act or experience, and this creates greater difficulty in communication. Would you want to comment on that?

DR. CALDERONE: First of all, I think a lot of people have the same stereotyped notion you have, Dr. Black, and that is that when you do sex education, you are going to be educating about the act. That is not what I mean by sex education or what I tried to convey. Obviously, eventually the anatomical terms will have to be used. I used them to this adult audience for a specific purpose, but this is not something that has to be emphasized when you discuss things with kids. You happen to deal with a high level bunch of kids to whom the word "sensitivities" and the word "relationships" are very familiar.

But I have here a letter from a very different kind of well-educated girl, who is a church-going girl, stands high in the community, high in her school, and has lots of friends. She says among a lot of other revealing and very sober and objective things, because she is not a way out girl at all, "If you have sex, you both will have a lot of fun. Sex is an active sport, more enjoyable than tennis or bowling."

What I meant when we were talking before, were the kids who said to me, the sensitive ones, "We are bothered by the kids who have intercourse under the piano in the Common Room. Our parents didn't prepare us for this. When we and our dates go out on a lovely moonlight night, right under that tree as we go out the door are three couples having intercourse. This bothers us."

This girl is not going to be reached by your sensitivities at all. My point is that we have to start a whole lot earlier because it is much too late both for this girl and for the mother who sent in the question about her freshman daughter.

It is too late to reach the freshman daughter because sex is a personal and private decision and, therefore, what we have to do is prepare our children young enough to make these personal and private decisions with full sensitivity. I agree with you on that, Dr. Black, but you can't start where you want to start. You have to start way back.

DR. SCHEIDLINGER: In all fairness to the mother who asked this question, I would plead that perhaps it is not too late. A single communication sometimes can carry a message of very great potential. Let us just imagine for a minute some possible dialogue between this mother and her daughter.

I am talking in outline, but suppose this mother would say to her daughter, "You know, I could never have asked this question of my own mother, and you know what—it scares the dickens out of me. I wasn't brought up at a time when one could talk freely about these things, and it even scares me more because you are my daughter and I love you, and I am afraid unless you stop to think through some of the things you talk about, you will be hurt, and I don't want you to be hurt. So let us at least talk. I know you will make the decision because you are going off to college and no-body will be there to watch. In fact, some of the colleges have now changed their rules and boys can have girls in their rooms. So I know you will make your decision. But at least let us talk over some of the pros and cons, some of the feelings involved."

Perhaps this mother will reach her daughter. If not, I have known of many young people who have made one mistake, and they needed to make this one mistake in order to learn that what mother has tried to convey really had some sense to it. And so I am somewhat optimistic that even then maybe it is not too late for a sincere dialogue, the kind of dialogue some of the morning speakers mentioned.

CHAIRMAN RABINOW: Another question we received, was what can a parent do should her daughter come and tell her that she is pregnant. Dr. Scheidlinger's comment to parents that children may make mistakes, just as they did, is terribly important to help parents anticipate these problems.

Some of the mistakes may be quite different. But what the children are looking for is, what does it mean when you make a mistake? They ask themselves, do I have parents who have the courage to live through this with me? Or are they only parents who we can come to when we feel happy?

One adolescent I knew said, "You know, I can't understand what this thing is that you parents have. All you want is for us to be happy." In a sense she is saying that *we* know there is more to life than just being happy. I think this is a reminder of how much we need to be tuned to the possibility that things will not always be as we hoped and planned for our children, and that even handling such a problem as an unexpected pregnancy may be a way of continuing sex education.

DR. BLACK: The function of the ministry, whether ethical or theological, results in our having such problems come to us. A family comes to us and wants to know what is right to do. Their eagerness, of course, is to protect this young person, that this shall not have been a mistake, they say, that might ruin a life.

In an ethical society or culture, it wouldn't. Now there are a few towns in this state where a girl can have a baby and be unwed and she can keep the baby and it is accepted, and there is no disgrace and nothing to be ashamed of about it. But in the middle-class community, even in liberal New York, I am not sure this is true.

Even with our absolute abortion laws, if you have money, you can pay and solve the problem that way if you want an abortion. But what this means emotionally to the particular young person we can't always know.

This year I had this kind of experience with one family in particular, who broke the law and paid a fortune. The doctor was unprofessional in that it involved a tremendous price, but it was done in one of the best hospitals. We still don't know the effect on the girl.

It is one thing to talk about a liberal position, but how then do you bring about a society where a person can make a mistake and mature through it, and would the people who believe in this be willing to liberalize the abortion laws as part of their liberalism?

DR. CALDERONE: I think that most thoughtful people now are beginning to realize that when people call me up, I say to them, "Look, the decision as to what will be done next should be a matter for the girl, the boy, and the four parents to sit down with a counselor about, because I honestly believe that few things are irretrievable in the world. Certainly the redemptive power of human beings to change and grow is enormous.

This can be a growing experience if it is handled right and not in a spirit of hysteria or panic—"Let us have the wedding quick," and a sixteen-year-old goes down the aisle with all of the accoutrements of a pretty marriage, the bridemaids and thrown bouquet, and a year later you have a divorce and a baby being brought up by a young child. This is a terrible, terrible solution in most cases.

I don't think that abortion is the right solution except, of course, in certain cases such as incest or rape or when there is a severe health threat to the child and mother.

In Sweden, a civilized nation, there are centers where the unwillingly pregnant mother can go and talk out her views and anxieties. Very often the solution she accepts is not abortion. I think this is something we have got to face as a society. The problem of the pregnant single girl could be a growing, learning experience with everyone protected, including the child who will eventually be adopted into a family willing and happy and ready to take care of it.

CHAIRMAN RABINOW: The last comment certainly points up the reason why there are no final answers: even when we achieve new and serious answers to the pressing problems of today, they raise other questions. I think it is well to take note that in Sweden and other countries where they feel they have conquered some problems that have to do with sexual relationships, they have created others.

I think finally that perhaps some of the answers will come from what Dore Schary suggested at luncheon: We may not be able to answer the large questions, but we have a responsibility to make an honest effort to answer the searching, immediate questions we face in our individual lives, and in our roles as professional people in our communities.

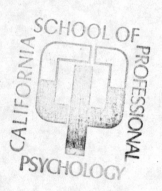